Belly Fat

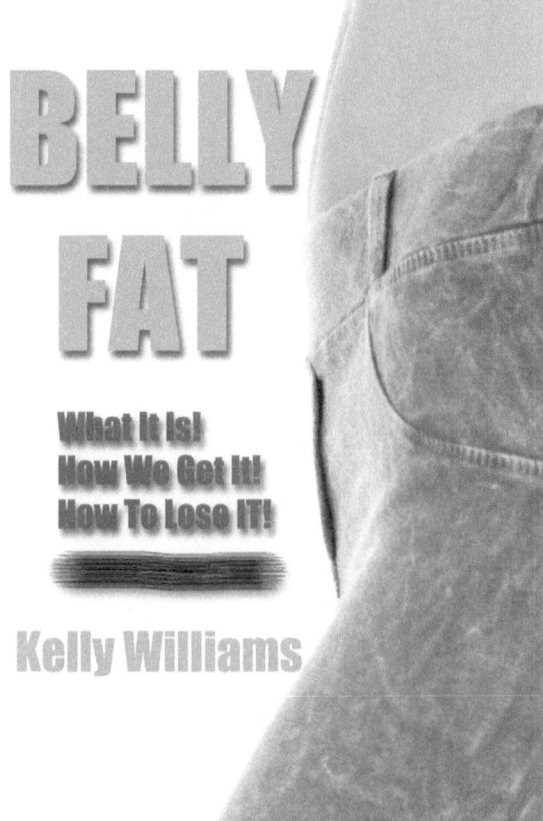

BELLY FAT

FAT

**What It Is!
How We Get It!
How To Lose IT!**

Kelly Williams

COPYRIGHT NOTICE

Also by Kelly Willaims

As The Days Go By: Step-by-Step Guide to a
Healthier and Happier Life

Disclaimer

The content provided in this book is for informational purposes only and is not a substitute for medical advice, diagnosis or treatment.

Belly Fat

<u>What It is!</u>
<u>How We Get It!</u>
<u>How To Lose It!</u>

Kelly Williams

What Is It?

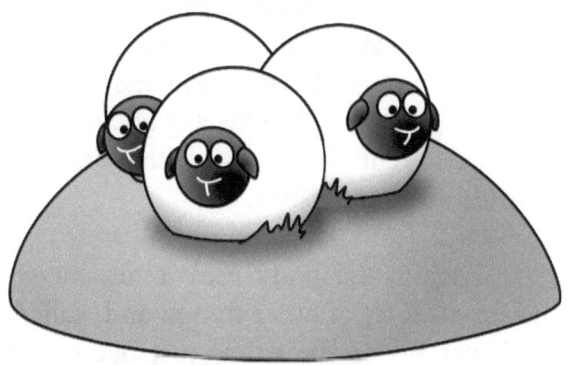

To understand what belly fat is one has to tackle fats in the first place. There are three kinds of fats to understand.

The *triglycerides* are the kind of fat that is in our blood, which the body needs for energy. When you have extras of this type of fat, then the body will keep it to use it "when" it needs in the future, instead of just getting rid of it. What are some of the places the body stores such fat? In the hips, for example, and your—you guessed it!— belly.

Unfortunately, if you have too much of this, then you're going to face health issues like heart disease.

Then, there is the *subcutaneous* fat. Its name in Greek means "beneath the skin" and basically gives you a mental image of where it is: beneath your skin tissue. It is literally right there. All over the body, it can be in different places, and the amount depends on your lifestyle.

Again, the body uses it for energy and for all sorts of other things, and, still, it won't get rid of the extras just because it likes to have the stuff around "just in case."

Finally, we have the *visceral* fat. Oh, this is a bad, bad fat. It is semi-fluid, and it hangs out between your organs in the abdomen. An excessive amount of this fat is known to lead to heart disease, diabetes, and a host of other health issues.

Oh, and yes, this is the "belly" fat you hear about (and probably fear).

But this fat is complicated.

"Visceral fat, or belly fat, has been linked to higher rates of heart disease and hypertension, for example," says the National Institute of Health, and then surprising that "subcutaneous fat that accumulates in the hips and thighs appears to offer some protection against chronic disease."

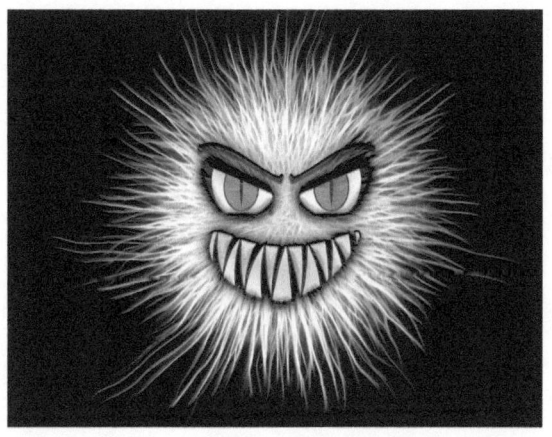

So, unfortunately, belly fat is not something that just sits on our bodies for curvy looks. Nor is it a "spare tire," as the old saying goes. No, it actually goes further and can destroy our health and can lead to our demise.

Next up, we ask and answer the question of … how do we end up with this?

How Do We Get It?

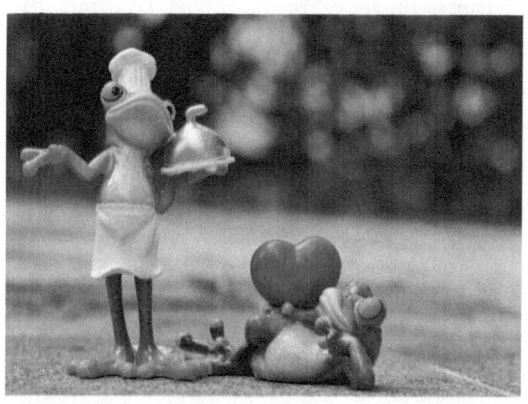

These days I think we all basically understand that there is an interaction between our genes and our environments. We understand that that interaction has a lot to do with how we feel, how we look, and how we behave.

Of course, scientists are continually discovering more ways to help us better understand this.

For example, in 2016 the National Institute of Health published a study that discovered about seven new areas of the genome linked to body fat distribution. The study, which included more than 18,000 individuals of European, African, Hispanic, and Chinese ancestry, was the largest ever to examine genetic variants across the genome and their association with ectopic fat, which accumulates in the abdominal area. The findings appeared in a December issue of the journal of *Nature Genetics*.

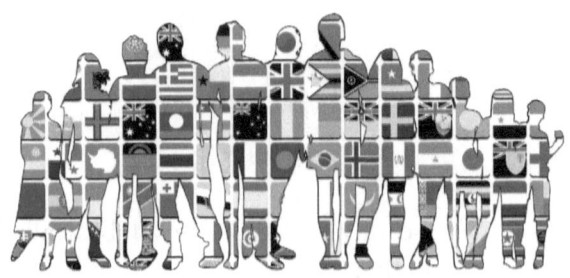

The researchers said that by identifying genes that are associated with ectopic fat, they can "learn more about the biological mechanisms that may influence individual differences in the risk for cardiometabolic diseases."

It also has to do with age, and somewhat gender as well. In 2015, folks at the Harvard Medical School said that as "people go through their middle years, their proportion of fat to body weight tends to increase — more so in women than men.

Extra pounds tend to park themselves around the midsection."

Although Harvard described the usual risk factors from belly fat to heart disease and diabetes, it said that in women it is "also associated with breast cancer and the need for gallbladder surgery."

Yikes.

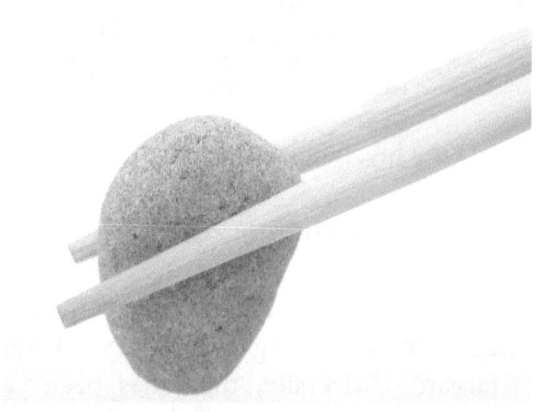

Another way we get it is through our food. When you intake more food than your body can use or discard, then you have extra stuff that can cause all sorts of things, including body fat, and especially belly fat.

It doesn't sound fair, but that is just how the body works. It has to do with our genetic background, our history, and our experiences—that the body doesn't just throw away the "garbage," as you'd like.

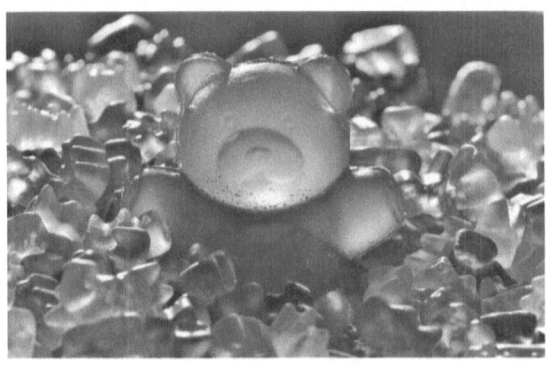

One big, bad wolf?

The sweet stuff.

During the past 30 years in the United States, according to Dr. Mary E. Choi of Harvard University, there has been "a marked increase in daily intake of fructose largely as a result of the introduction and widespread use of high-fructose corn syrup to sweeten beverages; however, we are beginning to recognize the not-so-sweet side of fructose."

You see it everywhere. Candy is so much cheaper than vegetables. So much is added to make it even "more" sweet. You're offered sweet stuff for celebrations, for sad moments, for even a visit to the doctor!

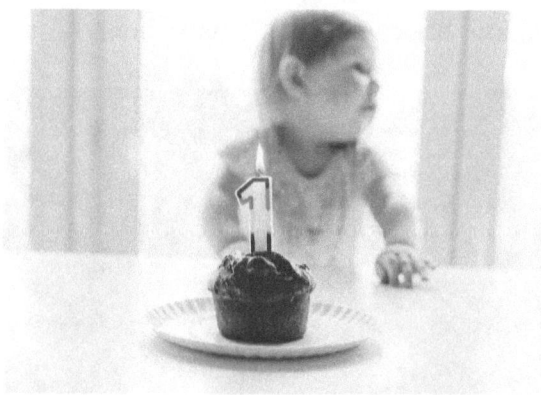

And for many of us, it starts from childhood. Sometimes, it starts before you can even have memories you remember as an adult.

"I have a picture of me with a cake as an infant," says a friend.

Of course, it is not coincidence that she loves cakes so much. She *knows* they are not good for her health.

She just can't help herself.

Another guilty group is alcohol.

Think about it, most of us don't even associate drinking "too much" with health issues. After all, every day after work, millions of people go to "happy" hour.

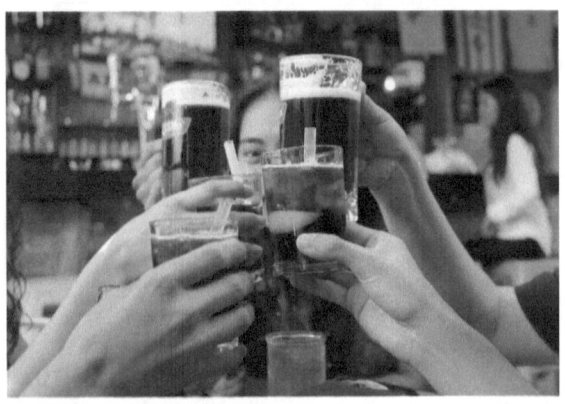

When they say "Beer Belly," don't think they are exaggerating.

One study, by researchers at the Lipids and Cardiovascular Epidemiology Research Unit of the Institut Municipal d'Investigació Me`dica in Spain, said that a "significant association of alcohol consumption with abdominal obesity and exceeding energy intake recommendations was found among men reporting consumption of more than 3 alcoholic drinks per day."

So, while bad food and alcohol are indeed cultural, there are also other factors.

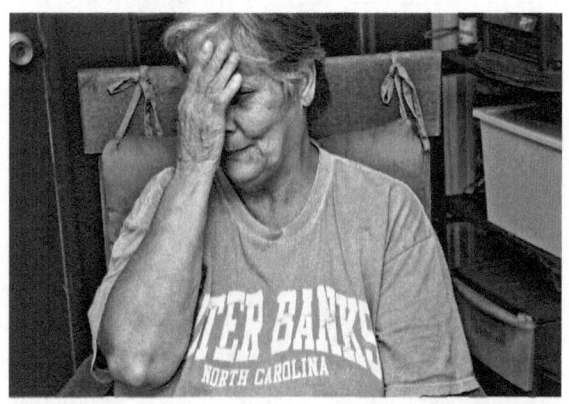

For the ladies, it's not just about genetics, food, or age.

Things like hormones, which can change or vary in any age group for a host of reasons, can also make a big impact.

"Many women also notice an increase in belly fat as they get older — even if they aren't gaining weight. This is likely due to a decreasing level of estrogen, which appears to influence where fat is distributed in the body," note folks at Mayo Clinic.

You know one of the rarely talked about reasons women develop low estrogen? Extreme dieting!

When you follow an extreme dieting, you're literally depleting your body fats—not just the "bad" ones but also the good!

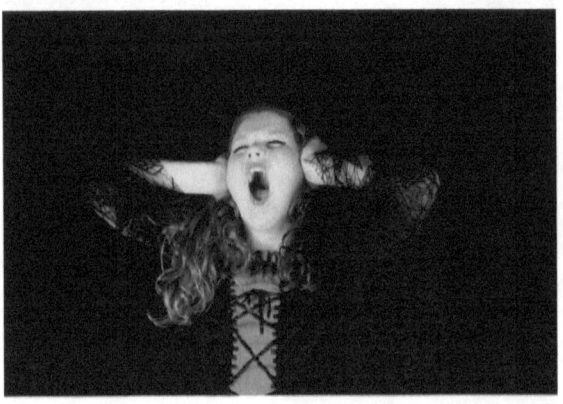

Finally, stress.

You just wake up and there is already stress. We can't really "escape" from all stress, but unnecessary often stress leads to hormone imbalances.

"Cortisol affects fat distribution by causing fat to be stored centrally—around the organs," notes Yale University, adding, "People with diseases associated with extreme exposure to cortisol, such as severe recurrent depression and Cushing's disease also have excessive amounts of visceral fat."

When your body is stressed, it secrets cortisol, which, as you see, is a nasty hormone.

Therefore, it is not just hormones you are running low of but also hormones that show up!

So, there are many causes. Next up, let's find out if you do have "it"?

Do I Have It?

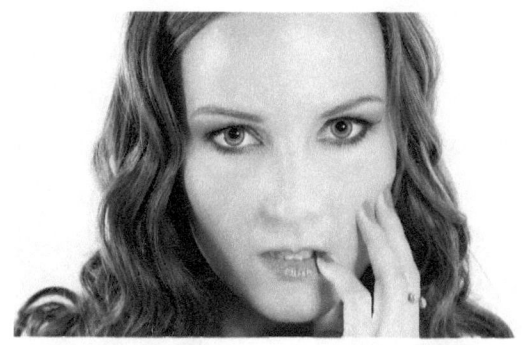

Now that you understand what it is and how we end up with it, the next part to adventure on is if you actually have belly fat or not. Are you really dealing with an issue, or is it just about being cute?

Grab a measuring tape.

If you don't have one, then make a quick run to the drug store and get yourself this important household item!

Once you have your measuring tape in hand, then you want to wrap it around your bare midsection. Measure the area immediately above your hips.

How many inches does it take to wrap it around you?

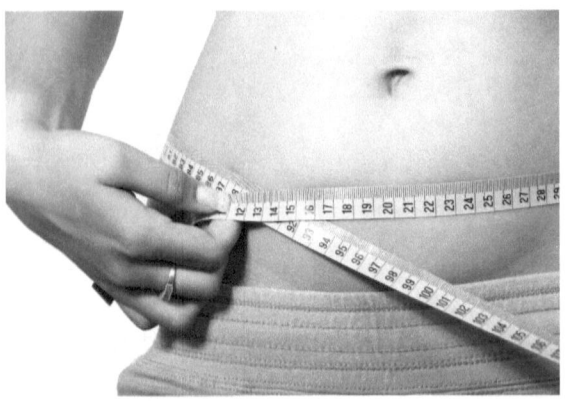

If you're a woman and it is more than 35 inches, then you're facing issues. If you're a man and it's more than 40 inches, then you're facing issues, too.

Simple as that.

Of course, your doctor can give you more detailed information. For example, your doctor will be able to tell you if there are health issues you're facing because of your belly fat or not by having you take a simple blood test.

Your doctor will also be able to help you understand your BMI or body mass index.

Next up, how do we get rid of it?

How To Get Rid Of It

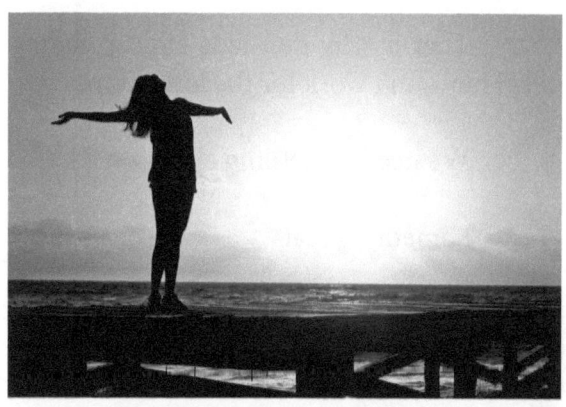

Getting rid of belly fat is not as difficult as you think it is. There really is only one simple formula to do this, and anything else is just a scam, and that "formula" is making a shift of lifestyle.

Note, I did not say exercise or food or anything else.

Why?

Because the real truth of the matter is that anything that is not a lifestyle change won't really change it. Those other things might lead to change for a brief moment or for a short-term, but you will end up with more than you started out with.

That is why diet fads end up fading out. They don't work for the long term.

We need something else.

Something real.

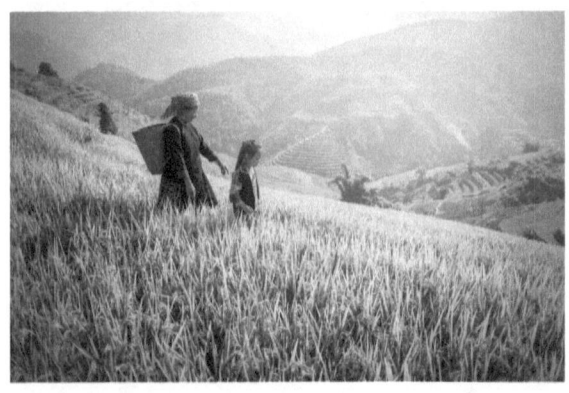

Think of it this way, our ancestors did not do diets. They lived and survived, and their entire focus was on how to get through the days.

So, what really changed?

Why are our lives so much unhealthier than, say, even thirty years ago, as Dr. Mary E. Choi from Harvard University pointed out?

Our lifestyle changed for the worse!

So, to win the battle with weight in general one has to really change the lifestyle to a healthier lifestyle.

Don't worry, it is easy.

Here are some ways to do it!

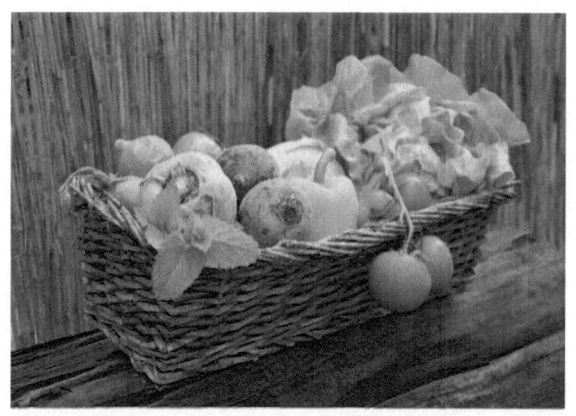

Eat Good Food:

In the case of fighting bad fat, the normal assumption is all about movements.

But did you know about the food?

Oh, yeah, the food you eat is just as important as what you do after eating it.

My suggestion?

Limit foods made by machines. Limit foods that are not real foods. If it can stay on the shelf for so long, what makes you think it is not going to sit in your abdomen?

Try eating *good* fats.

What are "good" fats?

Think of monounsaturated fatty acids, which are abbreviated as MUFAs.

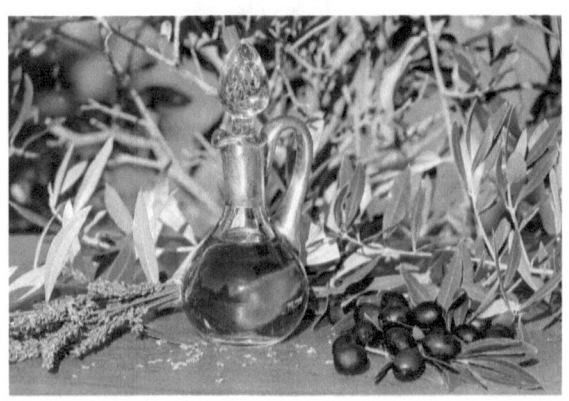

They are fatty acids. They have one double bond in the fatty acid chain, with all of the remainder carbon atoms being single-bonded.

So, what foods include these great good fats?

Mayo Clinic says foods like olives and olive oil, canola oil, nuts such as almonds or cashews or pecans and macadamias.

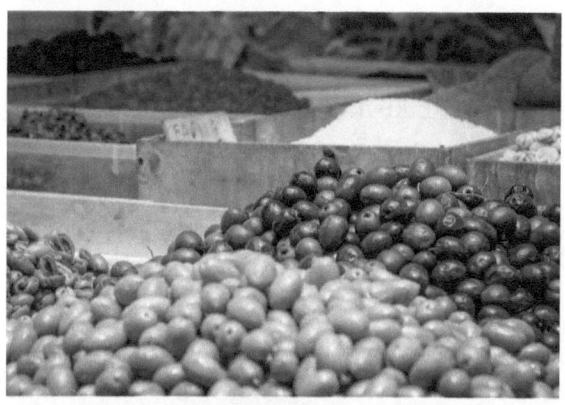

These are delicious foods!

Who wouldn't want to implement them in their daily diet?

Sadly, plenty of people.

Dr. Oz said that research from the journal of *Diabetes Care* found that "people who got roughly 25 percent of their total daily calories from MUFAs gained no visceral fat over the course of the study, while those who ate less MUFAs and more carbs added fat to their midsections."

So, as you can see, fighting bad fats is not as terrible as it sounds.

You can enjoy delicious food.

… Like milk!

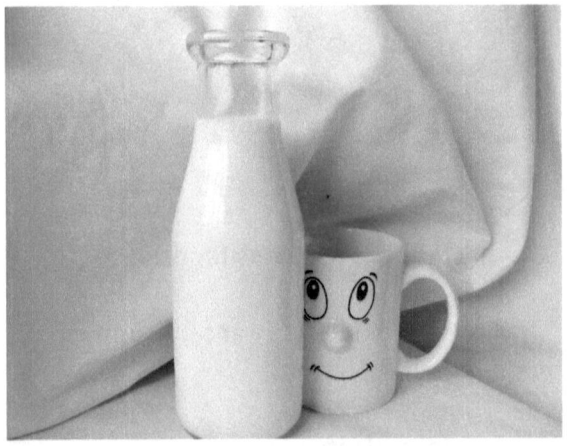

Calcium is another thing to pay attention to, as it is super essential for many reasons.

Researchers from the influential Shanghai Institute of Health Sciences found that calcium may be able to help with weight loss.

Their research says that calcium "plus vitamin D3 supplementation for 12 weeks augmented body fat and visceral fat loss in very-low calcium consumers during energy restriction."

My favorite motivating information about this is from Harvard: "Ninety-nine percent of the calcium in the human body is stored in the bones and teeth."

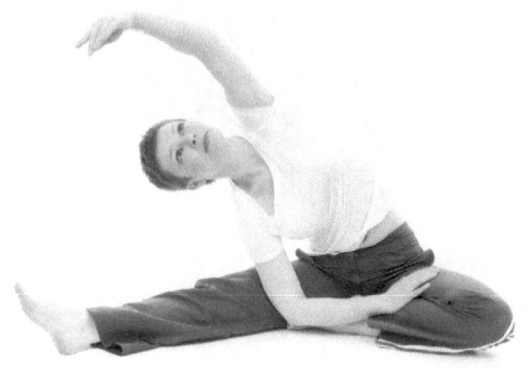

The general activities of calcium, regardless of where it is stored, are probably how it helps our fat loss.

Harvard University says that the body uses it for many things like "blood clotting, the transmission of nerve impulses, and the regulation of the heart's rhythm."

But, honestly, it does not matter what type of food you eat if you eat too much. If you overeat, you will be facing issues.

If you do the crime, you do the time.

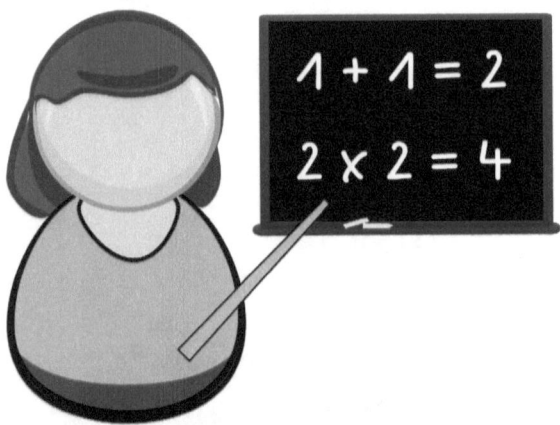

That is, if you eat a lot of food then you need to make sure the body either uses it or discards it.

How?

Move!

Human body is just really about the math. You eat + you move = what you ate is used for good. If you eat + don't move = what you ate is going to harm you in the long run.

Simple as that.

So, what do you do?

Before we get to the movement part, let me give you a sample of one day's worth of healthy eating.

Here it goes.

Morning

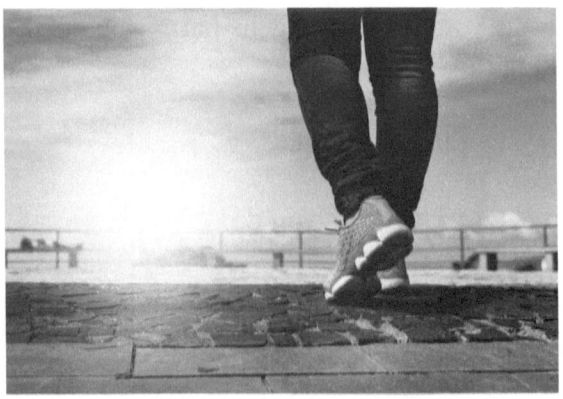

6am   You wake up, have a glass of water, and maybe you stretch. If you want to go for a walk, now would be a good time.

6:30   Now you're back. You can take a quick shower, or check your emails, or just catch your breath from your morning walk. However, don't wait too long because jumping into the shower will energize you.

7:30   You're out of the shower. You're starving! Why don't you start your beautiful day with a nice healthy breakfast? Let's say you have a cup of tea (or coffee, if you must), accompanied by a piece of healthy fruit (preferably banana), and some oatmeal mixed with yoghurt (preferably plain or Greek).

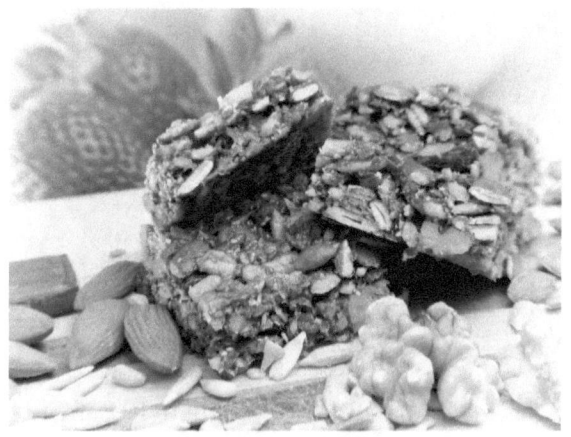

10am Let's say you're at work, or at home (and the kids are at school!), and let's say you're getting a bit hungry. You could wait for lunch, but you definitely want to munch on something. Let's do a morning snack! Grab something (small!) and enjoy it. I recommend a granola bar. Or perhaps an apple. Sometimes having an orange kind of "wakes" me up from my mid morning fatigue.

Afternoon

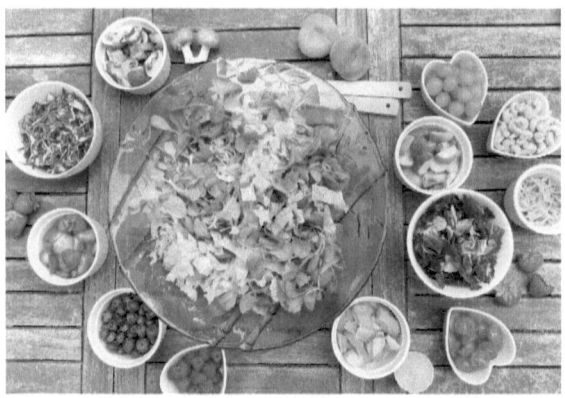

12:30 Oh, look at that! It's already lunchtime. Because you had a very healthy breakfast and mid morning snack, you could in *reality* continue your fabulous trend with a healthy lunch. I mean, look at that salad. You know it could be delicious! Of course, it would be so much better if you could, in fact, make it yourself. If you can't, then make sure to ask for the "Italian" dressing, instead of anything else that is heavy. If you must have a burger, at least keep the fries out.

3pm After 2 and ½ hours, you're ready for some snacking again. This time I will compromise with you. You have one cup of green tea and you can have something (small!) that is sweet along with it. I would, of course, recommend a piece of dark chocolate. If you don't want to have green tea, you can have something else and then you can't have that sweet thing.

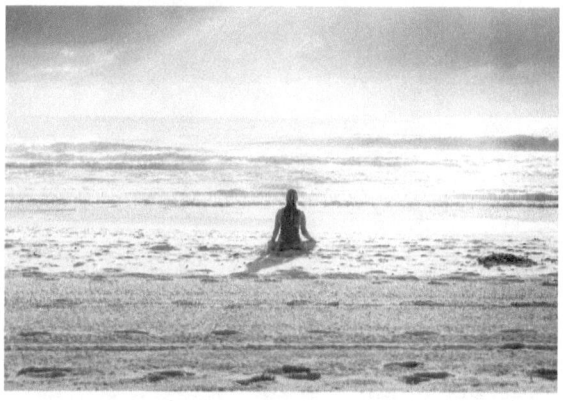

4:30   It is time to calm your mind. If you're religious, you can pray. If you're spiritual, you can meditate. If none of the above, you can take a quick nap that lasts less than 45 minutes. It's very important to do this step because it helps you to maintain a healthy balance of stress (yes, I know I used "healthy" and "stress" in the same sentence).

Evening

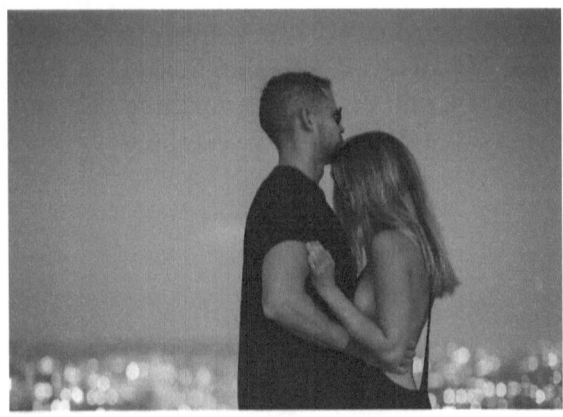

6pm   Dinnertime. For dinner, you can have a piece of protein. Let it be lean. Preferably chicken. Otherwise, get a nice piece of salmon. On the side you can have vegetables and brown rice. You could also have a glass of red wine.

8pm   Get happy. If you have a significant other, it is time to cuddle up to them and turn the world down. If not, it is time to watch something that uplifts you—perhaps your favorite primetime show.

9pm   It has been three hours since you ate. Now you could start getting ready for bed. You could have a nice bath. Or do your beauty routine. Take your time. Make sure to turn away from all digital products by now. That way, your natural sleep hormones will kick in.

10pm Bedtime. You want to make sure your room is comfortable. You don't want any kind of artificial lights. You also want to limit the amount noise. Good night.

Now let's talk about getting active.

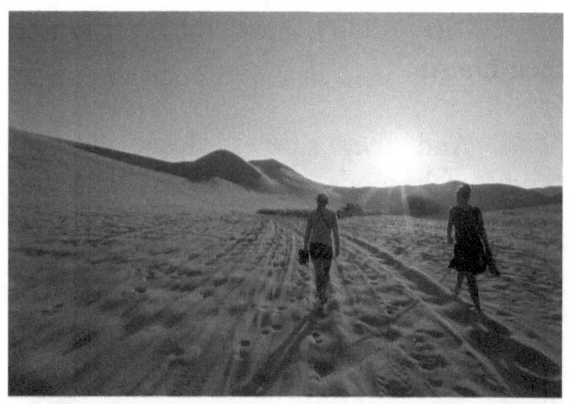

Be Active:

Our ancestors were constantly moving. Everything in their lives basically required they walk about it.

Remember, they worked hard for their food. They had to hunt or gather. They had to cook the foods from scratch.

They had to clean.

They didn't sit around and watch television all day.

They didn't have refrigerators.

They didn't have robots cleaning their houses.

And they sure as heck did not produce fake foods.

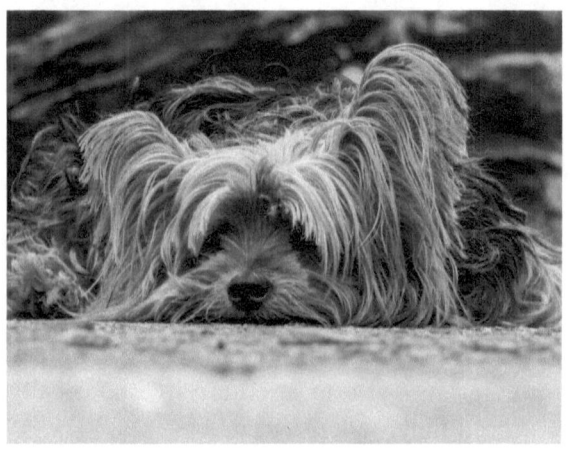

So, in the modern world, if you want to be in your cool house, and be in your car, or take the bus, or take the subway, or any of the other convenient ways that we live our lives, then you cannot go around moving intentionally.

So, you've got to be active.

Doesn't mean you have to go to a gym. You just need to move more.

"Walking counts, as long as it's brisk enough that you work up a sweat and breathe harder, with your heart rate faster than usual," says WebMD's Sonya Collins.

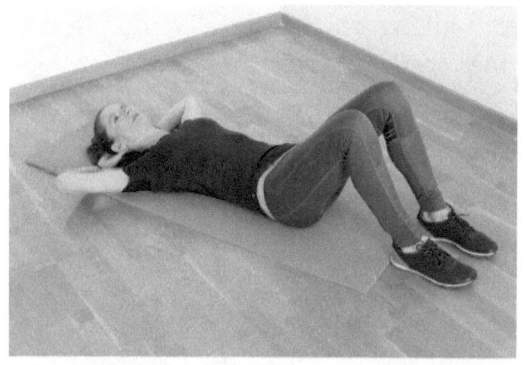

However, remember belly fat is not gotten rid of by crunches.

"Spot exercising, such as doing sit-ups, can tighten abdominal muscles, but it won't get at visceral fat," notes Harvard University.

Instead, they recommend, "regular moderate-intensity physical activity — at least 30 minutes per day (and perhaps up to 60 minutes per day) to control weigh."

1 hour out of 24 hours.

Easy!

However, if you can do more than just walking, it can really do wonders sooner, faster, quicker!

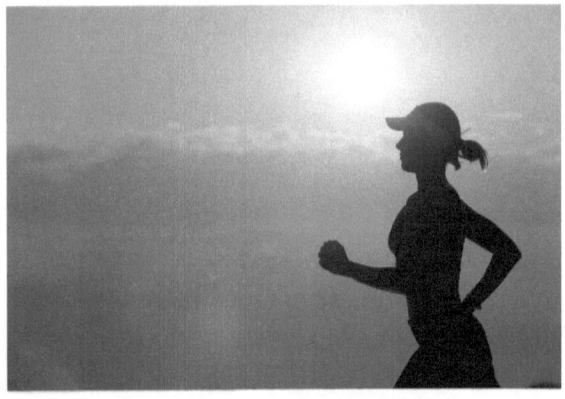

"A recent study from Duke University found that jogging the equivalent of 12 miles a week is enough to melt belly fat," note the good folks at *Women's Health*.

Don't let the big numbers scare you. Get your calculator out. Divide the overall miles by the days of the week, accounting for a day off.

So, 12 / 6 = to what?

Two miles per day.

Done.

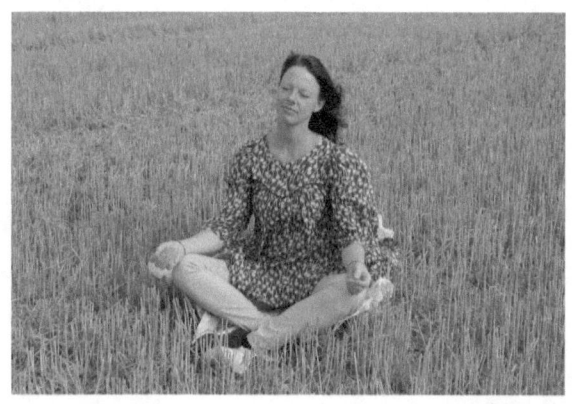

Relax:

No, really, you have to relax. Remember how I said when you're stressed your body secretes a hormone called cortisone, and the stuff is nasty?

Well, you've got to relax.

How?

There are really many ways!

"Any type of meditation will reduce anxiety and lower cortisol levels," notes *Psychology Today*'s Christopher Bergland, adding, "Simply taking a few deep breaths engages the Vagus nerve which triggers a signal within your nervous system to slow heart rate, lower blood pressure and decreases cortisol."

So, take a deep breath, hold it in the belly… Had to say it!

You know, almost every meditational guide tells their subject to "breathe deeply, let it go all the way to your stomach, hold it there," etc.

But, seriously, it calms you down and it gets rid of your belly fat. What could be better?

Sleeping and losing belly fat!

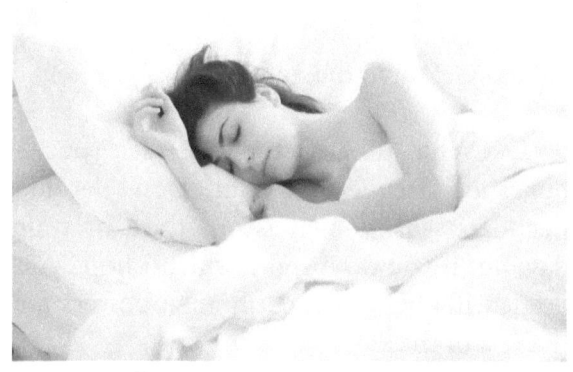

<u>Sleep:</u>

You probably have heard that sleep does wonders. Well, in this case it sure does!

"Not getting enough sleep does more damage than just leaving you with puffy eyes. It can cause fat to accumulate around your organs – more dangerous, researchers say, than those pesky love handles and jiggly thighs," wrote folks at Wake Forest University.

They had done a study that found there was a correlation between extremes of sleep – like not getting enough or getting too much – and visceral fat.

So, in a perfect world, you don't to sleep too long or too little.

Get on to the middle way.

What does that mean? Get your 8 hours of sleep every night. Don't let life negotiate with you. It is one-third of your day, but if you do it right, which I hope you do, it will give you super human powers for the rest of the day.

Okay, what is even better?

Breathing!

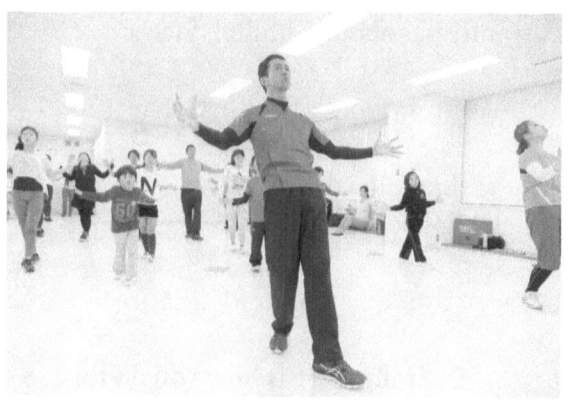

Breath Abs:

Okay, so there is a famous Japanese actor named Miki Ryosuke, who kind of by accident discovered something amazing.

"I was having back pain," he told the country's public television, "Then I was prescribed this in order to deal with my back pain. Then I realized my abs were getting great, and I was losing weight!"

What is this "Long Breath Diet" as it is called in Japanese?

See it for yourself.

There is a video on YouTube, which currently has about 5 million views:

https://youtu.be/9iJCGcDmygo

Book in the Amazon Japan store, which has about 44 reviews:

http://amzn.to/2qMCIE6

Basically, here is how you do this:

You stand straight, put your left leg a little forward and put the right leg back. You rest your body on the right leg, and you raise your arms to above your head while breathing in for three seconds.

Then, you stretch your hands out (as if you're inviting someone to a hug) and you put all of your muscles to work while exhaling for around seven seconds.

Easy as that.

Of course, with everything you learned about belly fat in this book, I think you understand by now that this is not the way to lose belly fat, but maybe it is for you.

What have you got to lose except your breath?

Go for it!

PERSONALIZE

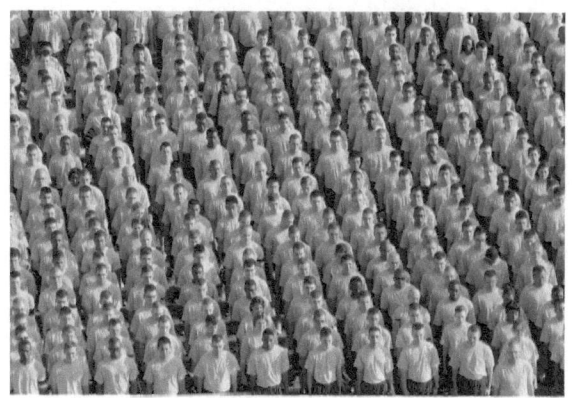

Our bodies are really complicated. One size does not fit all.

Although it is true we all have in common our basic make up, humans are diverse when it comes to the ways our bodies operate.

An African woman and a European woman could eat the same exact dish, yet their bodies would translate the incoming material differently.

Because, of course, as you have learned, there are many factors such as environment, genes, and even culture!

So, talk to your doctor. Ask him or her what should be your *real* body size—not the generic standard.

Don't accept the myth of medical standardization.

It is not true.

Do your research.

You're responsible for you.

Good luck!

About Kelly

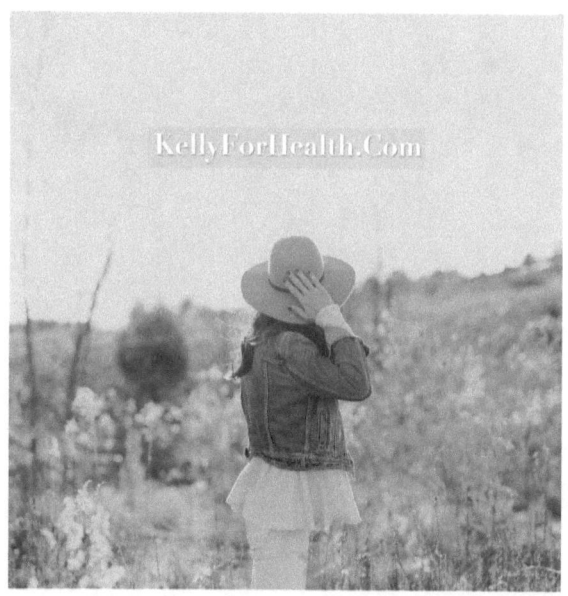

Kelly Williams is a writer who lives in the United States. Williams is the author of _As The Days Go By: Step-by-Step Guide to a Healthier and Happier Life_. The books by the author are based on own personal growth, following sound advice from experts at the top in their field, to live a better life. Visit her website: KellyForHealth.Com.